T0321178

RADIOLOGY
OF
DIABETES

.

RADIOLOGY OF DIABETES

B. E. Eyes, FRCR
Consultant Radiologist and Clinical Lecturer
Walton Hospital
Liverpool

I. A. MacFarlane, MD, MRCP
Consultant Physician and Clinical Lecturer
Walton Hospital
Liverpool

WKAP ARCHIEF

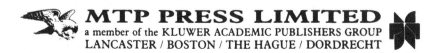

MTP PRESS LIMITED
a member of the KLUWER ACADEMIC PUBLISHERS GROUP
LANCASTER / BOSTON / THE HAGUE / DORDRECHT

Published in the UK and Europe by
MTP Press Limited
Falcon House
Lancaster, England

British Library Cataloguing in Publication Data

Eyes, B.
    Radiology of diabetes.
    1. Diabetes   2. Radiology, Medical
    I. Title   II. MacFarlane, I.A.
    616.4'620757   RC660

ISBN 0-85200-936-4

Published in the USA by
MTP Press
A division of Kluwer Academic Publishers
101 Philip Drive
Norwell, MA 02061, USA

Library of Congress Cataloging-in-Publication Data

Eyes, B. (Brian)
    Radiology of diabetes.
    Includes index.
    1. Diabetes—Complications and sequelae—Diagnosis.
2. Diagnosis, Radioscopic. I. Title.   II. MacFarlane,
I. A. (Ian A.) [DNLM: 1. Diabetes Mellitus—
radiography.   WK810 E97r]
RC660.E97   1986   616.4'62'0757   86-18619

ISBN 0-85200-936-4

Typeset by Blackpool Typesetting Services Ltd, Blackpool
Printed in Great Britain by Butler & Tanner Limited,
Frome and London

CONTENTS

PREFACE

This book is intended for those doctors in training who are involved in the management of diabetic patients e.g. physicians, surgeons, casualty staff, radiologists and general practitioners. It may also be of interest to medical students. We have given a brief outline of those conditions which may require radiology to help with decisions of management, but readers must consult a more comprehensive text on diabetes or radiology if further information is required.

ACKNOWLEDGEMENTS

We thank the following colleagues for their helpful advice and for donating radiographs used in this book:

Ann Ap-Thomas, Bernard Cohen, Mary Cunningham, David Harty, David Meek, G. Lamb, Trevor Smith, Robert Thompson and Graham Whitehouse.

INTRODUCTION

Diabetes mellitus is a common condition affecting 1–2% of the population in the United Kingdom. It is not a single disease, but a group of diseases, the common factor being a persistently raised blood glucose concentration. The major factor influencing the concentration of blood glucose in the body is the hormone *insulin* which is produced by the pancreas. If insulin secretion is reduced or if the action of insulin is impaired, blood glucose levels are raised.

Insulin deficiency is usually caused by autoimmune damage to the islet B-cells in the pancreas, probably initiated by an invading antigen (e.g. virus). This type of diabetes usually presents in childhood or young adults, but it is not unknown in old age. Other causes of insulin deficiency are pancreatitis, cancer of the pancreas, haemochromatosis (with iron deposition in the pancreas) and following pancreatic surgery.

However, in many diabetics raised blood glucose levels occur when relatively normal levels of circulating insulin are present. It is assumed, therefore, that the glucose intolerance in these patients is due to either mild impairment of insulin secretion or reduced sensitivity of tissues to insulin, or both. These patients are often overweight adults and in general show reduced numbers of receptors to insulin on target cells.

Rarely is diabetes due to the over production of hormones which oppose the action of insulin, e.g. cortisol (Cushing's syndrome); growth hormone (acromegaly) and catecholamines (phaeochromocytoma). In addition, corticosteroid therapy can precipitate diabetes, thiazide diuretics can reduce insulin secretion and pregnancy can impair glucose tolerance. Apart from these latter causes (endocrine, drugs, pregnancy) diabetes should be considered to be a lifelong disorder.

THE DIAGNOSIS OF DIABETES

When there is persistent hyperglycaemia glucose spills over into the urine (glycosuria), there is an osmotic diuresis and the patient may complain of thirst and polyuria. The diagnosis of diabetes is made by demonstrating hyperglycaemia, i.e. a blood glucose level of more than 11 mmol/l after food or greater than 8 mmol/l when fasting.

TREATMENT OF DIABETES

Once the diagnosis has been confirmed the objective is to reduce blood glucose concentration to normal, without producing troublesome hypoglycaemia. Some patients clearly have insulin deficiency and require insulin injections from the outset. These patients have severe symptoms (thirst, polyuria), weight loss and exhibit ketonuria, and without insulin they would progressively deteriorate, lose weight and die. These patients are diagnosed as having insulin-dependent diabetes mellitus or type 1 diabetes.

Most newly diagnosed diabetics, however, do not have a major weight loss or ketonuria. In these patients dietary treatment and weight reduction in the obese can reduce the high blood glucose levels, and are diagnosed as having non-insulin dependent diabetes mellitus or type 2 diabetes. Many will also require an oral hypoglycaemic drug in addition to a diabetic diet. However, in a significant number of type 2 diabetics oral drugs eventually fail to suppress hyperglycaemia, and they will then require insulin injections.

THE COMPLICATIONS OF DIABETES

After diagnosis, the majority of diabetic patients can be made free of hyperglycaemic symptoms if they are monitored carefully and their treatment is continually assessed. An important part of diabetic management is to detect and treat the chronic complications of diabetes which may subsequently arise (see Table 1). The evidence suggests that poor diabetic metabolic control and long duration of diabetes are associated with worse complications. Conversely good diabetic control may delay or prevent these complications.

Many chronic diabetic complications are secondary to damage to the structure of large and small arteries. Large arteries are damaged by atherosclerosis (macrovascular disease), whereas capillary lesions particularly affect the kidneys and eyes (microvascular

TABLE 1   THE COMPLICATIONS OF DIABETES

Acute	Hypoglycaemia
	Diabetic coma: Ketoacidosis
	Hyperosmolar state
	Infections
Chronic	Blindness
	Strokes
	Heart attacks
	Renal failure
	Autonomic and peripheral nerve damage
	Foot gangrene
	Infections

3

disease). Other chronic complications occur due to degeneration of peripheral and autonomic nerves (neuropathy). Macrovascular and microvascular disease and neuropathy are often seen together especially when diabetes is longstanding. It does not matter whether a patient is insulin treated or not, or what is the underlying cause of the diabetes, the same chronic diabetic complications can occur.

Hyperglycaemia and other metabolic disorders of diabetes can be present, with few or no diabetic symptoms, for many years. By the time diabetes is diagnosed many adult patients will already have developed complications. So-called 'mild' diabetics treated with diet or oral drugs can be lost to follow-up, only to present years later with an ischaemic, ulcerated foot and retinopathy.

Most diabetics are middle-aged or elderly and many take numerous tablets (e.g. for blood pressure, heart failure, etc.) in addition to oral hypoglycaemic drugs or insulin injections. In our hospital diabetic clinic, the average age is 58 years and the average duration of diabetes is 8 years, with over half of these patients showing medical problems other than diabetes (Table 2).

In addition to those conditions listed in Table 2 many have intermittent bowel disturbance, heartburn, urinary symptoms and dizzy spells. It must be remembered that 30% of these patients smoke cigarettes, despite being advised to stop. Unfortunately, over 40% of 'younger' patients (20–60-years-old) smoke and are thus voluntarily adding an extra cardiovascular risk factor.

TABLE 2   MEDICAL PROBLEMS OF PATIENTS ATTENDING WALTON HOSPITAL DIABETIC CLINIC

High blood pressure	22%
Calf claudication	18%
Eye trouble	17%
Bronchitis/emphysema	14%
Angina	12%
Previous myocardial infarction	9%
Leg/foot ulcers	6%
Peptic ulcer	5%
Stroke	5%
Neuritis	3%

THE CARE OF DIABETIC PATIENTS

The lifelong nature of diabetes and the occurrence of diabetic complications with time, leads to the involvement of many different specialists in the management of diabetes (Table 3). The care of elderly patients with severe diabetic complications is especially difficult and time consuming.

The hospital radiology department is frequently requested to help in the investigation and management of diabetics. Radiological

TABLE 3   WHO LOOKS AFTER DIABETICS?

Doctors
Diabetic clinic physician and junior doctors
Other physician specialists (renal, cardiovascular, neurology, geriatrician)
Orthopaedic and vascular surgeons
Ophthalmic surgeon
Obstetrician
General Practitioner
Accident and emergency doctors

   aided by:
Bacteriologist, chemical pathologist and radiologist

Nurses
(Out-patients, ward staff, liaison nurse, district nurse, health visitor)

Dietician
Chiropodist
Social Services
Pharmacist

procedures are usually requested in order to determine the presence and extent of chronic complications of diabetes. Occasionally they may help in the management of acute diabetic metabolic disorders and in determining the cause of diabetes. In addition, the radiologist has an important role to play in the monitoring of fetal development during a diabetic pregnancy.

PREPARING DIABETIC PATIENTS FOR RADIOLOGICAL PROCEDURES

When patients are referred for radiological procedures the request card should contain information as to the type of diabetes and the current diabetic treatment. The information may help the interpretation of the X-ray findings, but more importantly it will identify those diabetics who need special advice on how to prepare for specific investigations requiring starvation, purgation or fluid restriction (Table 4). These preparations may be hazardous in diabetics particularly those treated with insulin or oral hypoglycaemic agents, unless instructions are given to adjust their diabetic treatment.

TABLE 4   RADIOLOGICAL PROCEDURES REQUIRING PREPARATION

Radiological procedure	Preparation
Barium swallow meal Small bowel meal Oral cholecystogram Certain ultrasound scans	Starve from midnight
IV urography	Six hours fluid restriction
Barium enema	Low residue diet and purgation

Both general practitioners and hospital staff (consultant and junior doctors) are equally poor at mentioning diabetes on X-ray request forms. When diabetes is indicated it is often unclear and abbreviations are common, e.g. DM, IDDM, DM on tab, DM on INS. etc. The majority of doctors assume that patients will be instructed by ward nursing staff (in-patients) or the X-ray department (out-patients) on how to modify their insulin or oral drug treatment. Unless the appointment clerk specifically asks all out-patients about diabetes and its treatment, many diabetics will be instructed to starve or restrict fluid and receive no advice on how to modify treatment. Some intelligent patients will either alter their treatment appropriately or seek further advice, but many do not and become confused, particularly the elderly. The patients may or may not omit their insulin or oral drug on the day of the investigation.

Starving may induce hypoglycaemia which can cause irrational or aggressive behaviour or if severe, even coma. If the X-ray department is unaware that the patient is a diabetic treated with oral hypoglycaemic agents or insulin, chaos can result. Some insulin-dependent patients can rapidly develop ketosis if insulin is omitted for more than a few hours. Vomiting and acidosis with overbreathing can occur.

Patients referred for intravenous urography are normally instructed to restrict fluids beforehand. However dehydration is not advisable in diabetics as this may precipitate renal damage. Unfortunately, doctors commonly forget to mention diabetes on the request form for intravenous urography.

Recommendations for the management of diabetics treated with insulin or oral hypoglycaemic drugs are shown in Table 5.

It must be remembered that the responsibility for ensuring that diabetic treatment is adjusted to comply with the X-ray preparation rests with the referring clinician. If a patient does arrive starved and has taken his oral hypoglycaemic drug or insulin, a few spoonfuls of sugar dissolved in a small amount of water and swallowed should prevent hypoglycaemia.

TABLE 5   DIABETICS TREATED WITH INSULIN OR ORAL HYPOGLYCAEMIC DRUGS: MANAGEMENT DURING RADIOLOGICAL PROCEDURES

Starve from midnight
These patients should omit their morning insulin or oral hypoglycaemic. They should appear first on the morning list. Facilities should be provided for the patient to be given insulin or oral drug and breakfast

Fluid restriction
Patients attending for urography are usually fluid restricted and starved for 6 hours prior to the investigation. The diabetic should not be fluid restricted. Again he should appear first on the morning list and facilities provided for administration of insulin and breakfast. A low osmolar contrast agent, which is less nephrotoxic should be used

Low residue diet and purgatives
This preparation is complicated. Many insulin treated patients need to be admitted for 24 hours beforehand to stabilize the diabetes and to ensure adequate colonic preparation. If it is not possible to perform the enema in the morning an insulin and dextrose infusion should be given

---

THE CARDIOVASCULAR SYSTEM

CORONARY ARTERY DISEASE

Diabetes increases the risk of developing coronary artery disease, especially in women. Compared with non-diabetics there is a two-fold increased risk of myocardial infarction and mortality is greater. Recurrent infarction and heart failure are more common. The 5-year survival figure following the first myocardial infarct is only 20% compared with 50–70% in non-diabetics. This gloomy outlook may, in part, be due to disease of the myocardium.

PERIPHERAL VASCULAR DISEASE

Lower limb ischaemia due to atherosclerosis of the arteries supplying the legs leads to claudication, ischaemic rest pain and ulceration. Gangrene occurs five times more frequently in the diabetic compared with non-diabetics. Atherosclerosis is diffuse and involves distal as well as proximal vessels. This distal involvement is often untreatable with surgery. Medial calcification (Monckeberg's sclerosis) is often present in longstanding diabetics, especially those with neuropathy, resulting in unreliable measurements of ankle systolic pressure.

Arteriography is needed to decide whether arterial reconstruction is feasible. Angioplasty, using intraluminal balloons to dilate stenoses, may help those patients whose disease is unsuitable for surgery or those who are unfit for general anaesthetic.

CEREBRAL ARTERIAL DISEASE

Strokes are twice as common in diabetics than in non-diabetics and the prognosis is also worse in diabetics, 50% dying within a year. The indications for investigations (arteriography and CT scanning) in diabetics with transient ischaemic attacks or established strokes are the same as in non-diabetics.

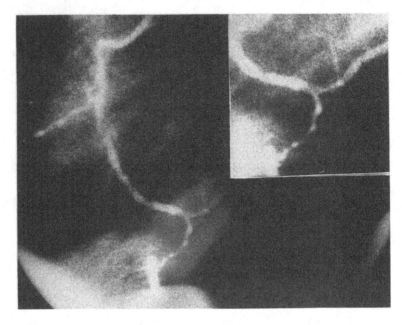

FIGURE 1   RIGHT CORONARY ARTERIOGRAM

This shows extensive irregularity of the right coronary artery due to atheroma. The enlarged inset shows the plaques involving the peripheral branches. This distribution of the lesions is common in diabetics

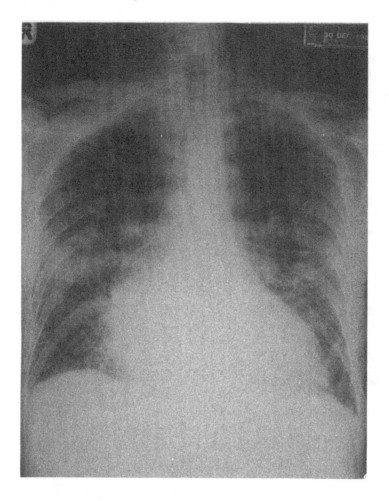

FIGURE 2   HEART FAILURE

The heart is enlarged. There is interstitial pulmonary oedema with Kerley lines A and B

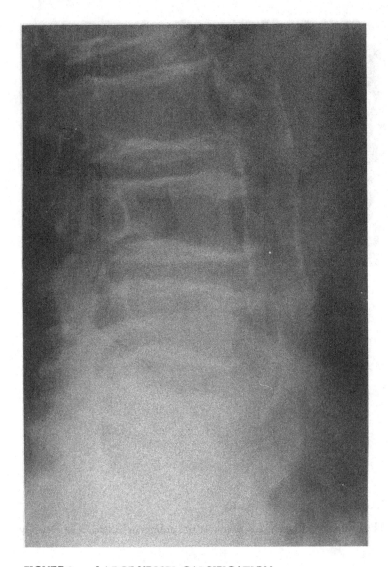

FIGURE 3   LARGE VESSEL CALCIFICATION

Lateral radiograph of abdominal aorta showing extensive atheromatous calcification. The calcification extends down into the iliac arteries

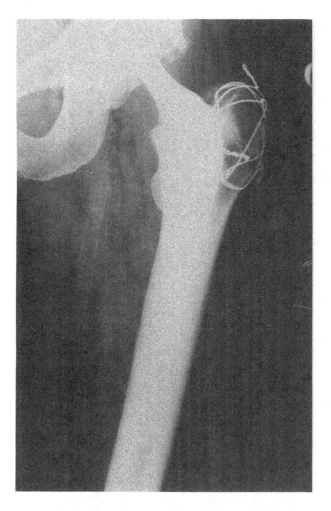

FIGURE 4   LARGE VESSEL CALCIFICATION

This shows heavy calcification of the 'cystic medial necrosis' type in the superficial femoral artery and also in the profunda femoris and its branches

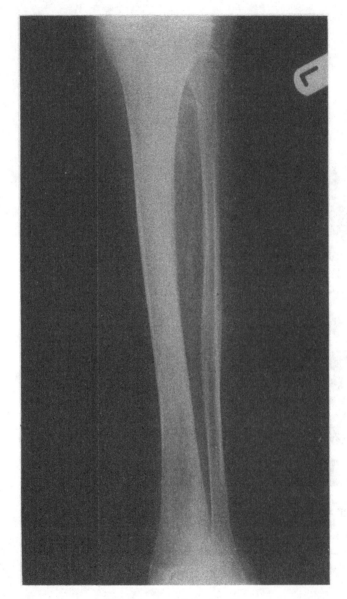

FIGURE 5   CALF VESSEL CALCIFICATION

Extensive calcification is shown extending down the tibial and peroneal
arteries

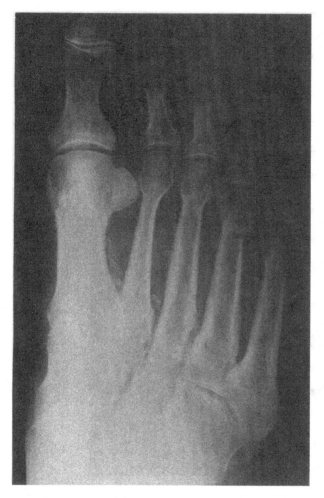

FIGURE 6   SMALL VESSEL CALCIFICATION

Typical inter-digital calcification in the plantar arteries

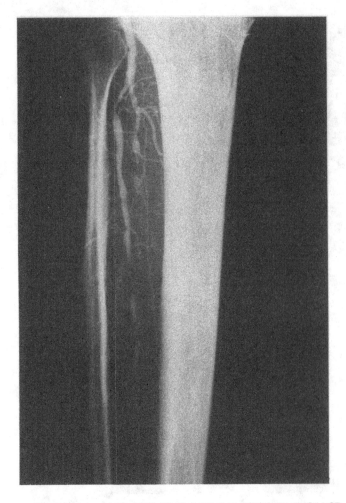

FIGURE 7   ARTERIOGRAM OF CALF VESSEL DISEASE

This demonstrates the typical diffuse and peripheral arterial disease with areas of occlusion and stenoses. This distribution of the disease make surgical correction difficult if not impossible

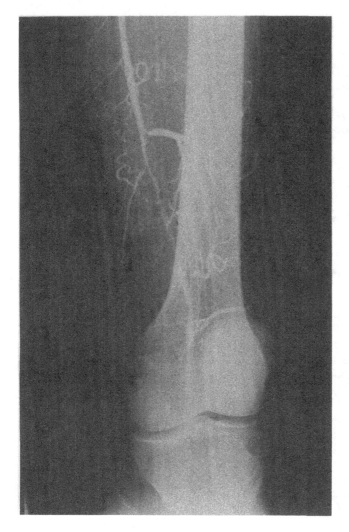

FIGURE 8   ANGIOPLASTY

Femoral arteriogram showing atheromatous plaques in the adductor canal narrowing the arterial lumen. Collateral vessels are shown around the stenosis reconstituting the popliteal artery

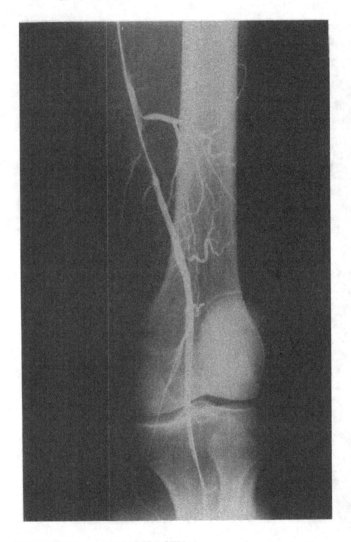

FIGURE 9   ANGIOPLASTY

A guidewire has been advanced into the popliteal artery to enable a balloon catheter to be placed across the stenosis

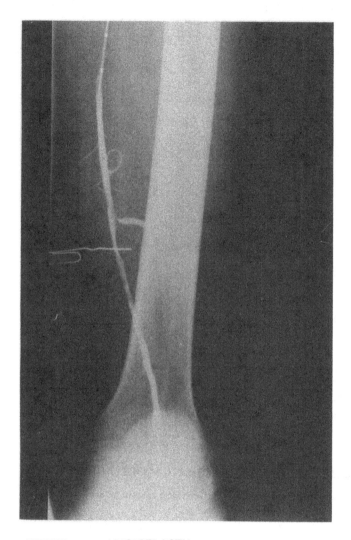

FIGURE 10   ANGIOPLASTY

The balloon has been inflated and the stricture dilated. A post procedural angiogram shows considerable improvement in the appearances. (The paper clip marks the area of atheroma during positioning of the balloon catheter)

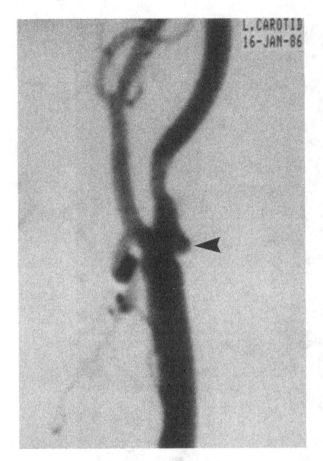

FIGURE 11   DIGITAL SUBTRACTION CAROTID ARTERIOGRAM

Atheromatous ulcer (arrowed) in the common carotid artery

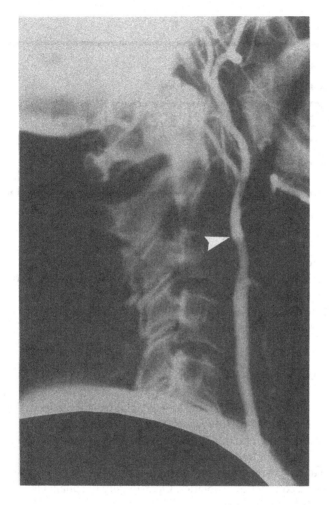

FIGURE 12   CAROTID ARTERIOGRAM

There is complete occlusion of the internal carotid artery due to atheroma.
The arrow shows the origin of the internal carotid

THE GASTROINTESTINAL SYSTEM

Visceral autonomic neuropathy is the most important cause of gastrointestinal problems in diabetics. Other mechanisms may also play a role: small vessel disease, abnormal blood glucose and electrolyte levels, increased susceptibility to infection and altered hormone production (e.g. insulin, glucagon).

OESOPHAGUS

Oesophageal symptoms (heartburn, dysphagia) usually occur in the presence of generalized peripheral neuropathy. Oesophageal motility is abnormal, and dilatation, delayed emptying and tertiary contractions can be found. Manometric studies may reveal weakened and infrequent peristalsis, increased spastic contractions and decreased contraction velocities. Occasionally dysphagia is associated with monilial oesophagitis.

STOMACH

'Gastroparesis diabeticorum' describes the atony and delayed gastric emptying in some diabetics. Other diabetic complications are usually present. Symptoms may include nausea, vomiting, heartburn, abdominal discomfort and bloating. However, it is often asymptomatic. Barium studies show gastric dilatation, reduced peristalsis, prolonged retention of barium and duodenal atony. Gastric bezoars may form. Irregular passage of gastric contents may lead to difficulties with diabetic metabolic control. If treatment with metoclopramide fails, surgical drainage procedures may be necessary.

SMALL INTESTINE

Small intestine dysfunction can cause diarrhoea. 'Diabetic diarrhoea' occurs in bouts, often at night, and is brown, watery and voluminous. Steatorrhoea is not present. Other causes of diarrhoea which must be excluded are:

(1) Metformin treatment
(2) Colonic neoplasm
(3) Inflammatory bowel disease
(4) Coeliac disease (probably increased incidence in diabetics)
(5) Pancreatic insufficiency
(6) Bacterial overgrowth
(7) Parasitic infestation

The cause of diarrhoea in diabetics is often unclear, and treatment is often empirical aimed at relieving symptoms. Antibiotic therapy is often used. Coarse, widened mucosal folds in the duodenum and small bowel are non-specific, and are seen in a wide variety of small bowel disorders.

LARGE INTESTINE

Large intestine motor abnormalities occur, usually in patients with peripheral neuropathy. Constipation can result but a colonic malignancy must always be excluded. Treatment may include high fibre diet, stool softeners, laxatives and metoclopramide.

ANAL SPHINCTER

Anal sphincter dysfunction occurs in longstanding diabetics and can cause faecal incontinence.

BILIARY TRACT

Gallstones and cholecystitis are more common in the diabetic population with abnormalities of lipid metabolism probably contributing to stone formation. However, gallbladder dysfunction secondary to neuropathy may also play a role. Large gallbladders which contract poorly after a fatty meal may occur. Poor visualization of the gallbladder during an oral cholecystogram may be due to prolonged gastric retention of the cholecystographic media.

Emphysematous cholecystitis, a mixed aerobic and anaerobic infection, occurs more frequently in diabetics. Gas is seen in the gallbladder lumen and occasionally in the gallbladder wall. Gangrene of the gallbladder and perforation are serious complications in diabetics, and the underlying cause may be arterial insufficiency.

PANCREATIC DISEASE

Pancreatic disease may cause diabetes (pancreatitis, carcinoma, cysts, or pseudo cysts). In chronic pancreatitis diffuse calcification outlining the pancreas is seen in the retrogastric space.

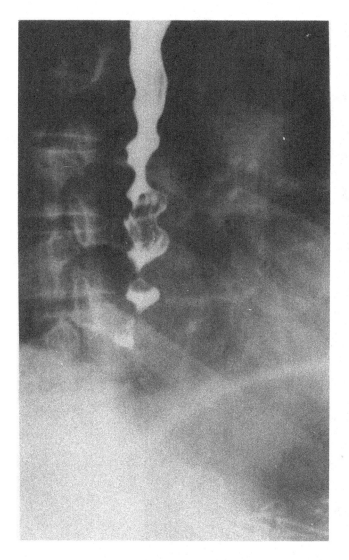

FIGURE 13   TERTIARY OESOPHAGEAL CONTRACTIONS

Oblique single contrast view of lower oesophagus showing 'corkscrew' appearance typical of tertiary contractions

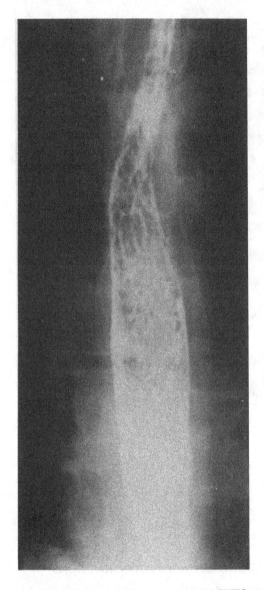

FIGURE 14   MONILIAL OESOPHAGITIS

Double contrast view of lower oesophagus showing multiple filling
defects due to monilial colonies

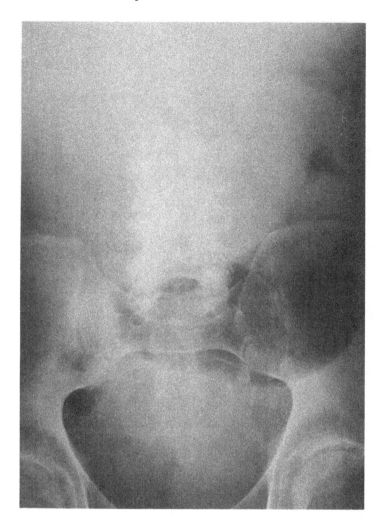

FIGURE 15   GASTROPARESIS DIABETICORUM

Markedly distended stomach after a 12 hour fast (supine film). Air and food residue fill the stomach. Barium studies showed a poorly emptying stomach with an atonic duodenal bulb and no pyloric obstruction. Peristalsis is infrequent or completely absent

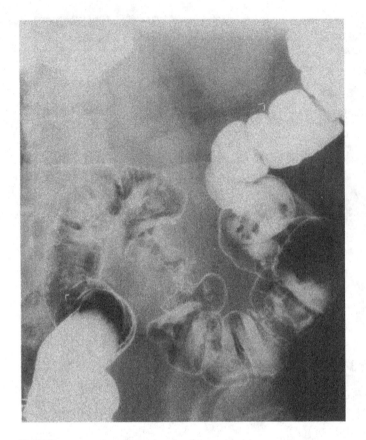

FIGURE 16   CARCINOMA OF THE COLON

Barium enema showing the typical 'apple core' appearances of a sigmoid colon neoplasm. Large bowel neoplasm must always be considered in diabetics with diarrhoea

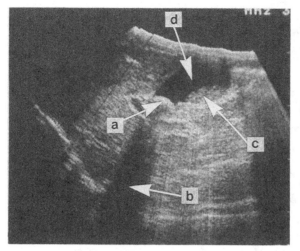

FIGURE 17   GALLSTONES

Ultrasound of the gallbladder demonstrating a calculus in the fundus of the gallbladder. The typical acoustic shadow beyond it is well demonstrated. The further opacity within the gallbladder not casting an acoustic shadow is due to biliary sludge. a = calculus, b = acoustic shadow, c = biliary sludge, d = gallbladder

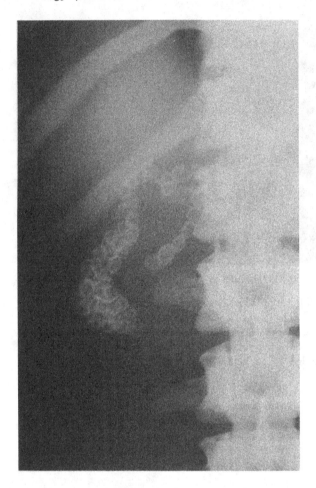

FIGURE 18   GALLSTONES

Plain film of right upper quadrant showing multiple opaque calculi in the gallbladder, cystic duct and probably down into the common bile duct

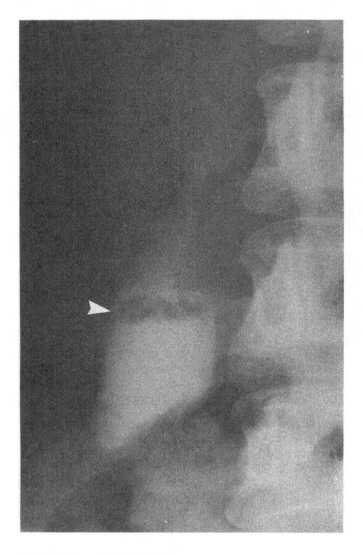

FIGURE 19   GALLSTONES

Erect film during an oral cholecystogram showing multiple radiolucent calculi (arrow) floating on the opacified bile

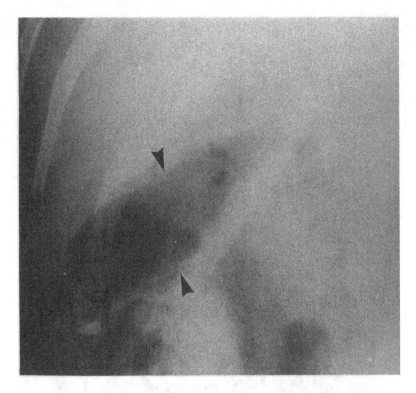

FIGURE 20   EMPHYSEMATOUS CHOLECYSTITIS

Supine view of right upper quadrant showing the gallbladder distended with air and air in the wall of the gallbladder (arrowed) due to infection with gas forming organisms

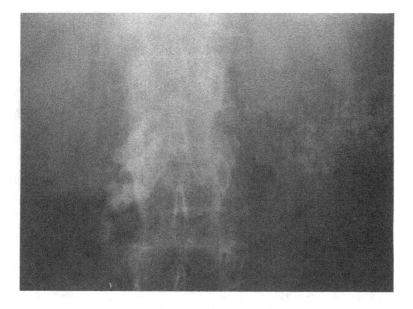

FIGURE 21   CHRONIC PANCREATITIS

Antero-posterior view of upper abdomen showing extensive pancreatic calcification involving the head, body and tail of the pancreas

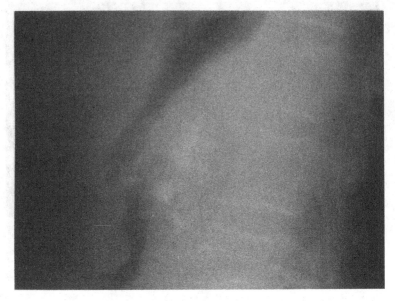

FIGURE 22   CHRONIC PANCREATITIS

Lateral view of upper abdomen showing enlarged calcified pancreas displacing the body of the stomach anteriorly. (The unusual appearance of the lower lumbar vertebra is due to an artifact)

THE KIDNEY AND RENAL TRACT

Diabetics have a 17-fold higher risk of renal failure than non-diabetics and in younger patients it is one of the commonest causes of death. Early in the course of insulin dependent diabetes the glomerular filtration rate is increased. Glomerular growth occurs and the kidney enlarges. Capillaries in the glomerular basement membrane then become thickened and the glomerulus is replaced by deposition of glycoprotein material. Kidney damage is made worse by ischaemia due to thickening of the renal arteries, hypertension and renal tract infections.

Intravenous urography is often requested in diabetics. Fluid restriction should be avoided in patients with impaired renal function or acute renal failure may result. In chronic renal impairment the renal tract is poorly visualized and the kidney size is variable.

Urinary tract infections are probably more frequent in long-standing diabetics (particularly women). Diabetic kidney tissue may be more susceptible to infection and autonomic neuropathy leads to a poorly emptying, atonic bladder with infected, static urine. In acute pyelonephritis, urography is usually normal but occasionally a large poorly functioning kidney is seen. In chronic pyelonephritis calyceal clubbing occurs due to fibrosis and scarring.

Infections can be severe and cause the renal papillae to slough (papillary necrosis). A poor papillary blood supply may be important in the development of papillary necrosis. In the early acute stages there is some shrinkage of the papilla leading to widening of the calyceal cup and local decreased function. Later, function improves and contrast enters clefts in the necrotic papilla.

Calcification can occur and the papilla appears as a triangular, calcified area. Necrotic papillae may detach giving rise to a 'ring' appearance. An obstructive uropathy may develop if a detached papilla enters the ureter. In chronic cases the kidneys appear atrophic.

Emphysematous pyelonephritis is caused by infection with gas forming organisms. Gas bubbles are seen in the renal pelvis and calyces, and can also appear in the bladder (cystitis emphysematosa).

Calcification of the spermatic tract (vas deferens, ampullae and seminal vesicles) in the absence of inflammation and stricture, is highly suggestive of diabetes. Usually the calcification is limited to the intrapelvic portion of the tract but can extend into the testicle.

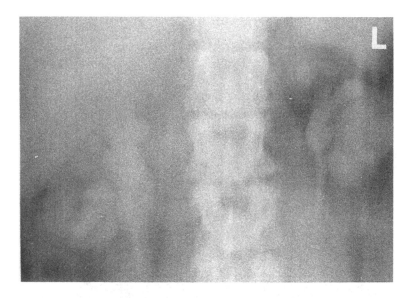

FIGURE 23   CHRONIC PYELONEPHRITIS

Intravenous urogram showing clubbing of the calyces in shrunken scarred kidneys. There is considerable loss of renal cortical substance

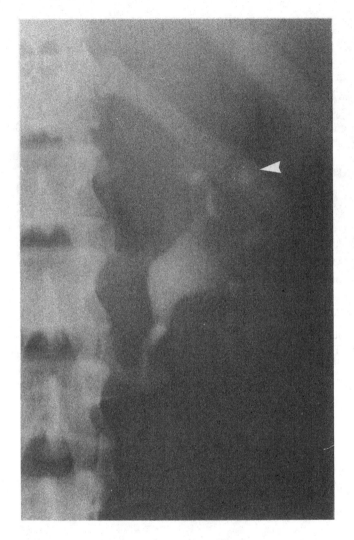

FIGURE 24   EARLY PAPILLARY NECROSIS

Early changes shown in the upper pole on a 15 minute IVU. The classical 'ring' shadow (arrowed) due to a separated papilla is shown

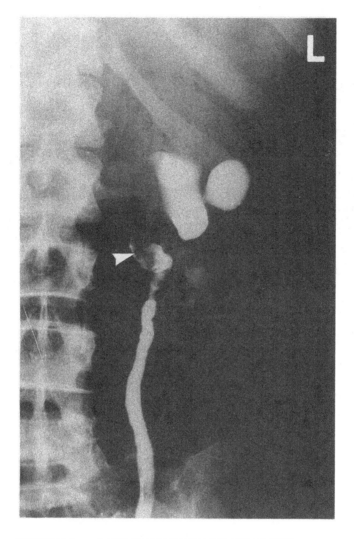

FIGURE 25   LATE STAGE PAPILLARY NECROSIS
(same patient as Figure 24, 2 years later)

Retrograde pyelogram showing a filling defect obstructing the pelvi-
ureteric junction due to a sequestrated papilla (arrowed). Gross clubbing
of the visible calyces is shown due to advanced papillary necrosis

41

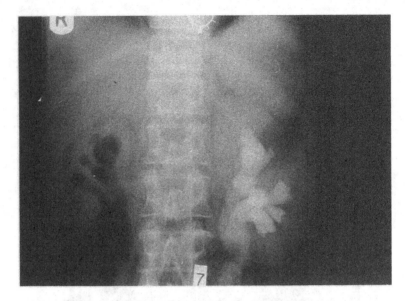

FIGURE 26   EMPHYSEMATOUS PYELONEPHRITIS

The right pelvicalyceal collecting system is shown to be filled with air produced by gas-forming organisms. The kidney is small and scarred due to chronic pyelonephritis

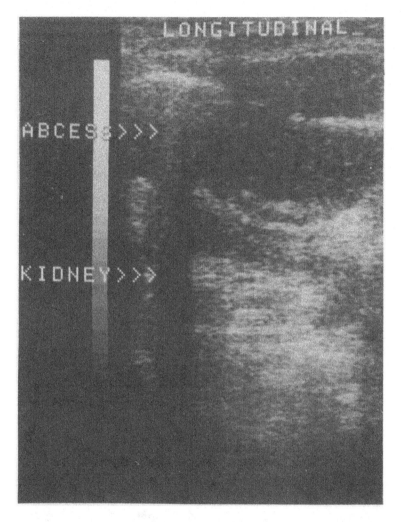

FIGURE 27   PERINEPHRIC ABSCESS

Longitudinal ultrasound scan showing a perinephric abscess collection
lying posterior to the kidney. This was successfully drained under
ultrasound control

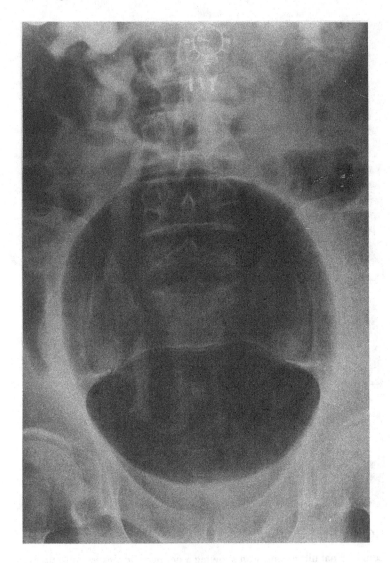

FIGURE 28   EMPHYSEMATOUS CYSTITIS

30 minute film of an intravenous urogram showing gross distension of the
bladder by gas. This patient was later shown to have a neuropathic
bladder

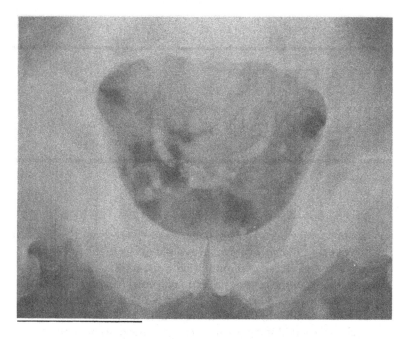

FIGURE 29   CALCIFIED VAS DEFERENS

Extensive vas deferens calcification. This can occasionally extend down into the testicles

DIABETIC PREGNANCY

When pregnancy occurs in a diabetic every effort should be made to achieve perfect diabetic control to avoid damage to the fetus. The patients treated with diet or oral drugs must start insulin injections. The wellbeing of the fetus is linked to placental function. Vascular impairment may lead to a small, scarred placenta and fetal growth retardation. Stillbirth, toxaemia and hydramnious can occur.

High maternal blood glucose levels cross the placenta and stimulate fetal insulin secretion. This may lead to excessive fetal growth and large birthweight infants who are prone to the respiratory distress syndrome.

There is an increased risk of congenital malformation in the fetus when maternal diabetic control was poor at the time of conception. The most clearly associated malformation is the caudal regression syndrome (femoral hypoplasia with agenesis of lower vertebrae). Other skeletal malformations are seen in addition to cardiovascular abnormalities. Fetal ultrasound measurements provide an assessment of placental size and fetal abnormalities and are also an index of fetal growth.

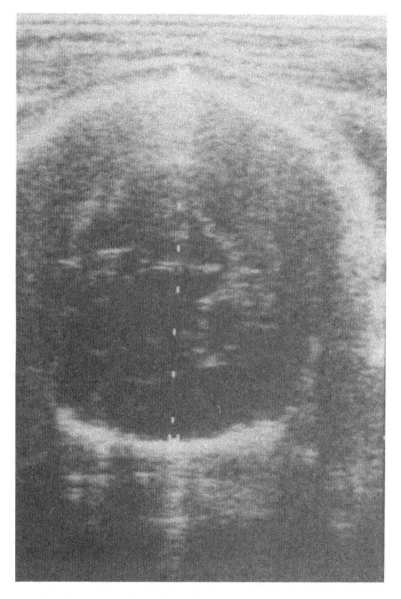

FIGURE 30   FETAL ULTRASOUND (1)

Transverse scan through head. Gestational age judged by the scan = 33
weeks 1 day

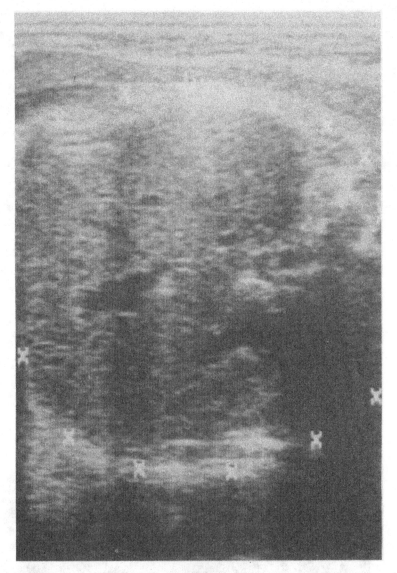

FIGURE 31   FETAL ULTRASOUND (2)

Transverse scan through the abdomen of the same fetus as Figure 30 at umbilical vein level. Gestational age judged by the scan = 36 weeks 4 days. This discrepancy in the gestational age as judged by the abdominal scan indicates visceromegally

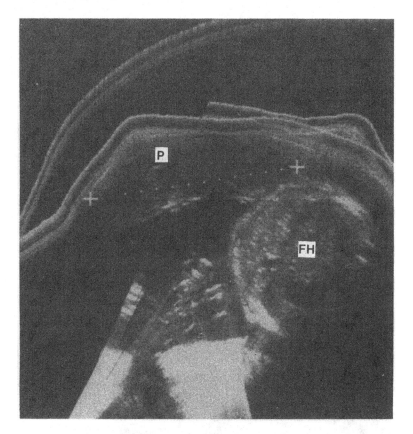

FIGURE 32   PLACENTAL ULTRASOUND

Ultrasound scan showing the placenta situated anteriorly. Placental volume calculations can be obtained from these scans and hence predictions of placental function can be made. (P = placenta; FH = fetal head)

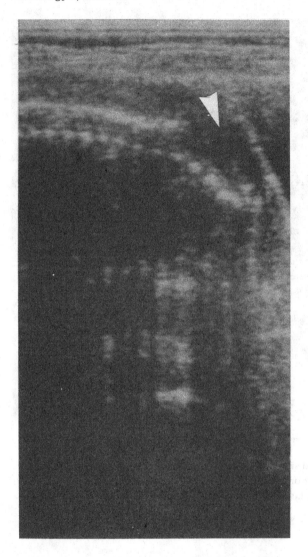

FIGURE 33   FETAL ULTRASOUND

Longitudinal scan of the fetal spine showing a defect posteriorly due to spina bifida (arrowed)

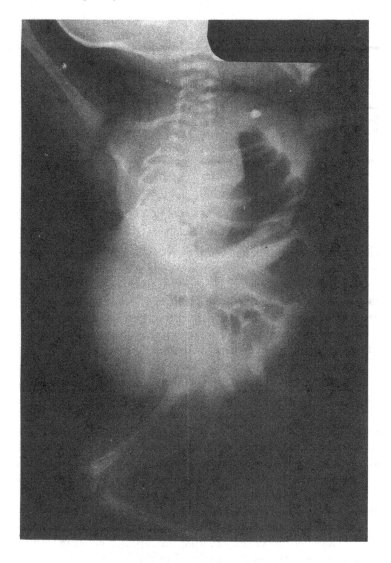

FIGURE 34   CAUDAL REGRESSION SYNDROME

Stillborn fetus with gross lower thoracic lumbar and sacral developmental anomaly. The caudal region of the spine has failed to develop

THE NEUROPATHIC FOOT

The foot of a diabetic can develop a variety of disorders secondary to peripheral neuropathy, peripheral vascular disease or both. Ulceration and gangrene occur more frequently in patients who have poor diabetic control, wear ill-fitting shoes and fail to have correct chiropody for difficult nail cutting, corns and callosities. Established foot lesions cause great disability, prolonged hospital admissions and sadly, often end with amputation.

Peripheral neuropathy results in sensory loss and sympathetic nerve damage. Blood flow in the neuropathic foot is increased, leading to excessive warmth and distended veins on the dorsum. This may be due to arterio-venous shunting resulting from sympathetic denervation. Sympathetic nerve damage can also cause structural damage to peripheral arteries and this may be the reason why medial vascular calcification develops. Foot deformities occur, particularly a 'claw foot' due to muscle weakness. Neuropathic foot ulcers develop at sites of maximal weight bearing, commonly the heads of the metatarsals and over the tops of the toes. Excessive keratin production leads to callous formation. Patients are unaware of callosities because of sensory loss, and repeated pressure from walking and ill-fitting shoes lead to ulceration.

A Charcot joint (neuropathic joint) can develop in diabetics with neuropathy. Minor trauma, such as tripping, may result in an acutely swollen, erythematous foot. Serial radiographs may then show progressive changes; fracture, osteolysis, fragmentation, new bone formation, subluxation and finally complete joint disorganization.

Occasionally severe peripheral oedema due to neuropathy can develop. This may be related to the high blood flow and arterio-venous shunting resulting from sympathetic nerve damage.

Infection in the diabetic foot is a major problem particularly when underlying bones and joints are involved. Progression of sepsis can be alarmingly rapid. Gas, due to gas forming organisms, may form in the tissues and this will show on the X-ray.

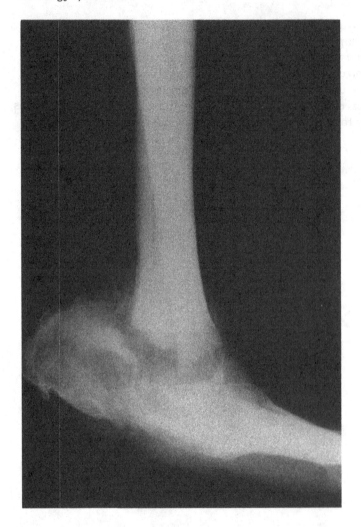

FIGURE 35   NEUROPATHIC ANKLE JOINT

There is complete disruption of the ankle mortice and tarsal bones. There
are bone spicules in the soft tissues and sclerotic changes in the tarsal
bones

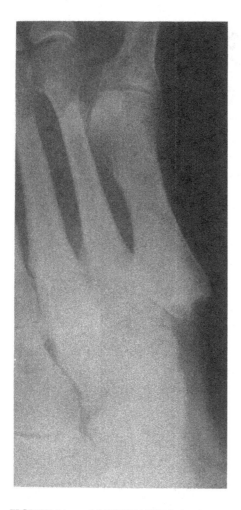

FIGURE 36   NEUROPATHIC CHANGES IN THE TARSUS

This advanced case shows marked sclerosis and loss of joint space between the tarsal bones. The medial cuneiform has been surgically removed

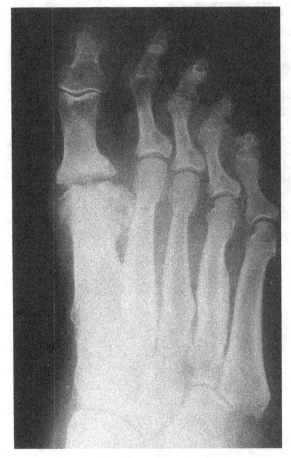

**FIGURE 37   NEUROPATHIC FIRST METATARSO-PHALANGEAL
               JOINT**

Irregularity of the articular surfaces of the first metatarsal and proximal
phalanx of the hallux is demonstrated. There is sclerosis and evidence of
fragmentation

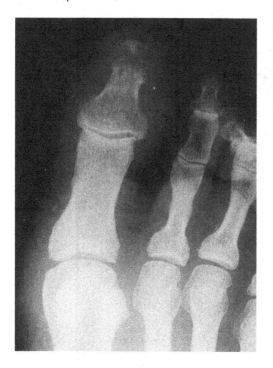

FIGURE 38   EARLY INFECTIVE CHANGES IN TERMINAL
PHALANX OF THE HALLUX

There is soft tissue swelling over the terminal phalanx. Destructive
changes are shown in the terminal tuft due to osteomyelitis

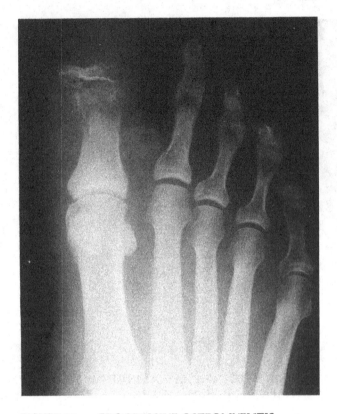

FIGURE 39   PROGRESSIVE OSTEOMYELITIS

Progressive destructive osteomyelitis almost completely destroying the
terminal phalanx and extending across the interphalangeal joint to the
proximal phalanx

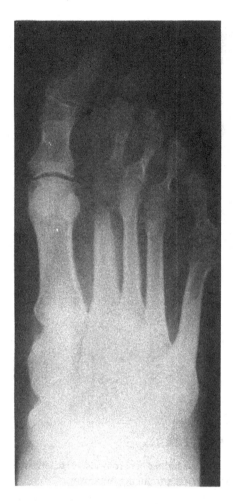

FIGURE 40   INFECTION

Osteomyelitis of second metatarso-phalangeal joint. Faint arterial
calcification is shown. There is destruction of the head of the second
metatarsal and base of the proximal phalanx of the second toe with
periosteal reaction along the metatarsal shaft

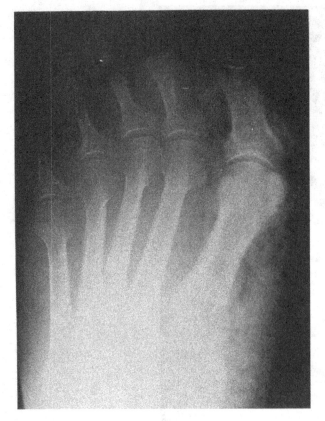

FIGURE 41   SOFT TISSUE INFECTION

Destructive changes are shown in the hallux. There is also extensive gas in the soft tissue due to infection with gas producing organisms

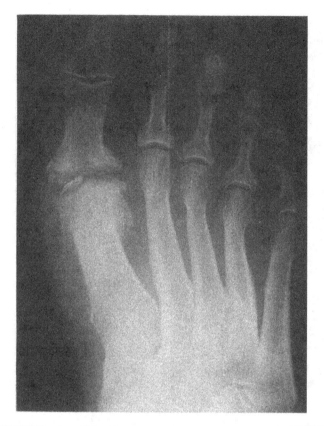

**FIGURE 42   COMBINED OSTEOMYELITIS AND NEUROPATHIC
CHANGES**

Irregularity and sclerosis around 1st metatarso–phalangeal joint due to
neuropathy. There is also a sequestrium in the metatarso–phalangeal joint
due to superadded infection and osteomyelitis

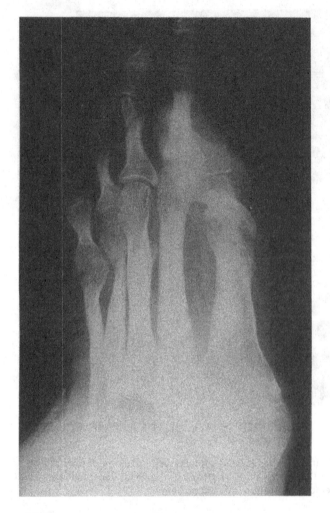

FIGURE 43   LONGTERM SEQUELAE

The tarsal bones are disrupted due to neuropathy. There is evidence of previous osteomyelitis in the first metatarso–phalangeal joint

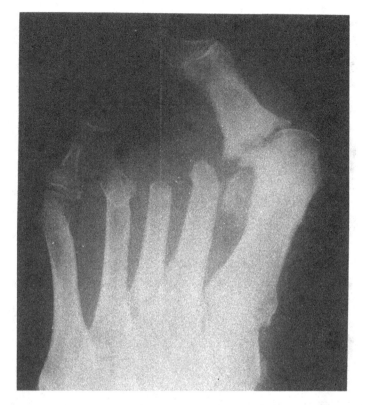

FIGURE 44   LONGTERM SEQUELAE OF NEUROPATHY, INFECTION AND ISCHAEMIA

The foot of a longstanding diabetic who has had 2nd, 3rd and 4th toes amputated due to ischaemia. There are neuropathic changes in the 1st metatarso-phalangeal joint

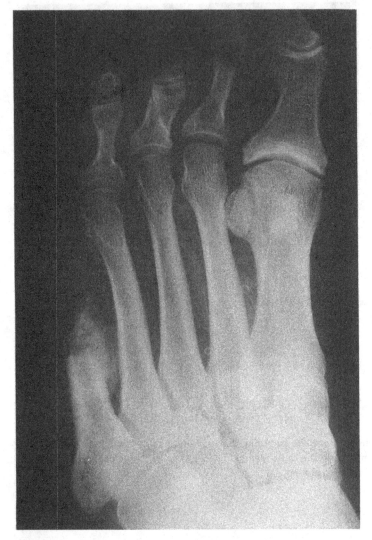

FIGURE 45   RESIDUAL OLD INFECTION AND ISCHAEMIA

Interdigital vessel calcification is shown. The distal half of the fifth
metatarsal has been amputated due to gangrene and infection

CONNECTIVE TISSUE ABNORMALITIES

Connective tissues (skeleton, joints, periarticular structures) are affected by diabetes. Many changes are seen but they can be divided into:
- (1)   Reduced bone density
- (2)   Inappropriate deposition of connective tissue.

(1) Osteoporosis
Poorly controlled insulin dependent diabetics are at risk of generalized osteoporosis. Insulin deficiency leads to net bone loss and bone turnover appears to be reduced. Osteoporosis can lead to hip and vertebral body fractures.

(2) New bone formation
Non-insulin dependent diabetics seem to be prone to inappropriate deposition of bone in certain sites. Ankylosing hyperostosis of the spine (Forestier's disease) is well recognized and may be detected in the investigation of back pain. New bone formation also occurs elsewhere: hyperostosis frontalis interna, calcification of pelvic ligaments, osteitis condensans ilii and occasionally around the hips, knees and wrists.

(3) The joints
Diabetes is the most common cause of neuropathic joints. The neuropathic foot has already been discussed. Some studies have shown an increased prevalence of osteoarthrosis in young and middle-aged diabetics which started at an earlier age and was more severe than in non-diabetic controls. There is no convincing evidence that diabetics are more prone to gout or pyrophosphate arthropathy than the normal population.

There are a number of clinical syndromes with pain and sometimes swelling of articular and peri-articular structures which probably occur more frequently in diabetics, i.e. adhesive capsulitis of the shoulder, shoulder–hand syndrome, fore-foot osteolysis and transient osteolysis of the hip and knees. Overlying vasomotor changes are common and joint mobility limited. There may be increased excretion of calcium and hydroxyproline and increased uptake of bone seeking isotopes. The natural course is spontaneous recovery but fibrosis and contracture can occur. Radiological changes of 'spotty' or diffuse osteoporosis are usually late developments.

Poorly controlled diabetics are prone to skin infections and foot ulceration is a common problem. Recently a condition resembling scleroderma, involving both the skin and peri-articular tissue has been recognized (diabetic cheiroarthropathy). Insulin-dependent patients may develop tight, waxy skin, tenosynovitis and restricted joint movement, principally over the palms of the hands. Other associations include the carpal tunnel syndrome and Dupuytren's disease.

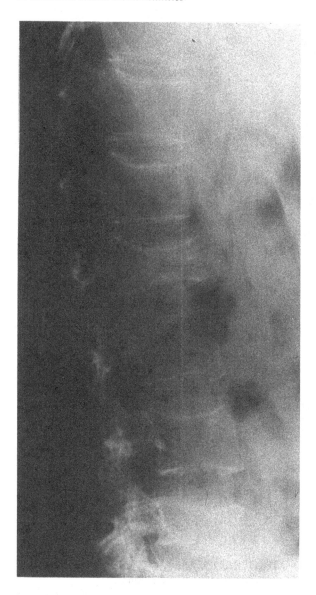

FIGURE 46   OSTEOPOROSIS

There is generalized osteoporosis in the lumbar spine in a 21-year-old diabetic girl. The 1st lumbar vertebra has collapsed due to demineralization

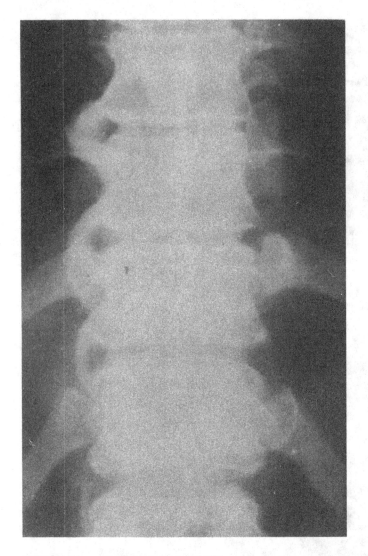

FIGURE 47   FORESTIER'S DISEASE
(A.P. view of thoraco–lumbar junction)

Gross osteophyte formation and vertebral ankylosis. Usually the anterior
parts of the vertebral body are affected with less marked changes laterally.
Massive bars of new bone are demonstrated. Typically the vertebral body
outline can still be seen

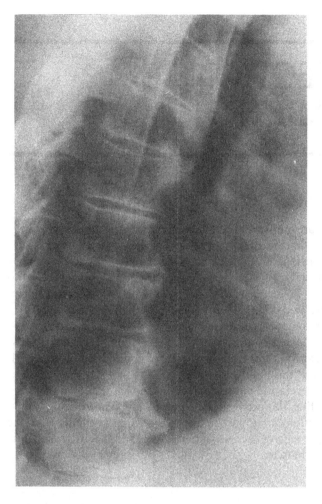

FIGURE 48   FORESTIER'S DISEASE

Lateral view of lower thoracic spine demonstrating the large anterior osteophyte formation and ankylosis

INFECTIONS IN DIABETES

Diabetics are more prone to infections, and infection is more likely if blood sugar control is poor. Several of the severe infections that may arise in diabetic patients have already been discussed (emphysematous cholecystitis and pyelonephritis, perinephric abscess, foot infections). Tuberculosis was once a common and serious problem in diabetics and occurred more frequently than in non-diabetics. Fifty years ago tuberculosis was a common cause of death but improved diabetic control (particularly insulin injections), effective screening and anti-tuberculous drugs have considerably reduced the prevalence of this infection.

Several severe and unusual infections such as pseudomonas external otitis, rhinocerebral mucormycosis and necrotizing soft tissue infections occur particularly in diabetics. The latter is characterized by extensive necrosis of the skin, subcutaneous tissues and underlying muscle.

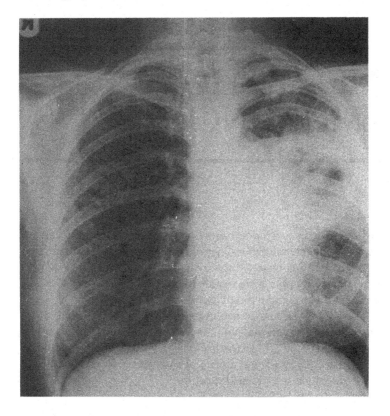

FIGURE 49   TUBERCULOSIS

Soft shadowing and consolidation is shown in the left upper lobe and apical segment of left lower lobe. Extensive cavitation is also demonstrated. The appearances are typical of advanced tuberculosis

METABOLIC
EMERGENCIES

Hypoglycaemia is a major hazard of insulin treatment but can also occur in patients taking oral hypoglycaemic agents. Diabetics in hypoglycaemic coma are often treated in hospital casualty departments and a number have sustained injuries from car or work accidents, burns and hypoglycaemic convulsions.

Ketoacidosis occurs in insulin-dependent patients. Severe vomiting and abdominal pain may occur. The stomach can be large and distended with a succussion splash. These symptoms and signs may misleadingly suggest a surgical emergency. Severe vomiting can however, cause oesophageal rupture.

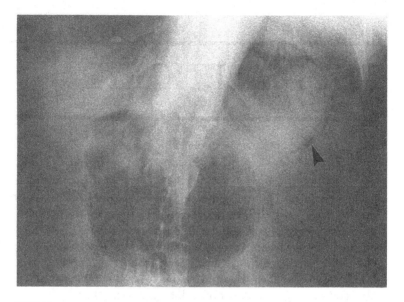

FIGURE 50   GASTRIC DILATATION

Supine antero-posterior view of upper abdomen showing a distended
stomach with air in the gastric wall in the fundal region (arrowed). Air is
forced into the gastric wall by repeated severe vomiting in ketoacidosis

THE DIABETIC EYE

Diabetic retinopathy is the commonest medical cause of blindness in the Western World. Vitreous haemorrhage is the great danger from proliferative retinopathy, and half the patients with this disorder are blind within 5 years unless treated with laser photocoagulation. Fluorescein angiography can demonstrate abnormal retinal capillaries, micro-aneurisms and leaking from microvascular abnormalities. Ultrasound of the orbit has prognostic value by its ability to distinguish between simple vitreous haemorrhage, haemorrhage with bands and haemorrhage with retinal detachment. In addition vitreous changes before and after surgery can be followed.

INDEX